Fancy New Products

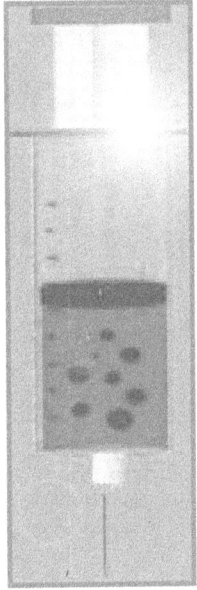

Stephen C. Rusbarsky, MPH, CIC, CSSGB

ISBN: 9781699942222

DEDICATION

This book is dedicated to all who are dedicated to the safety and care of patients. Also, everyone who strives to be better; to learn more; to achieve his/her goals. These people are the reason this book is written. Never stop caring, never stop helping others, and never stop learning.

Stephen Rusbarsky, MPH, CIC, CSSGB

Table of Contents

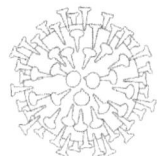

Introduction

I like to think of the job of an Infection Preventionist as a bunch of "P"s.

As in, we deal with People, Policies, Procedures, Places, and Products. If you are more creative than I am, I'm sure you can think of even more. "Products" is one of the most complex categories to deal with (probably because it's so closely-related to the behavior of people). In any given day, you may be presented with situations such as:

"These gowns are too hot"

"These new gloves aren't rated for the chemo drug I work with"

"We need to standardize our cleansing cloths (as in, get rid of all but one product); do we need to tell the nurses?"

"Can we use alcohol disinfectant caps on peripheral IVs? Can we put them on our Foley sampling ports?"

Is antimicrobial soap better than regular soap? Is foam better than liquid? Do I need to use a lotion after washing? Where should we place the new soap dispensers?

"We want a different product than the rest of the hospital. Can we just order what we want?"

There are probably about ninety-five more comments that could be added to the mix. And all are – more or less – valid points which need discussing. It is easy to get burned out or frustrated with products, and even easier to allow *product creep*…as in, give someone an inch and they take a mile, or in this case, give one unit a special product, and expect to see it in half the hospital several months from now. The intent of this book is to delve into situations, scenarios, and content which will strengthen your understanding of products as they relate to your position as an Infection Preventionist.

First, we start with the people who bring us the products. **Sales Representatives** are employees of a company whose job it is to *interpret* a product – how it is used, how it can help, and the science that shows that it works well. Often, in a healthcare setting, there are many people who must look at a product before it is brought in. For example, the IP doesn't care much about cost – he or she considers the product from the standpoint of "will it *prevent* infection or will it *promote* infection?" And, although someone with the money in your organization will care about the safety aspect, they are more concerned with the cost. A nurse might be mostly concerned with whether it'll make her or his job easier to care for a patient. Sales

Representatives should know that each person must review it with his/her peers (which can take time). The rep should be willing to go through the steps that a facility needs to take in order to bring a well-vetted product through the doors. Just as with any person in general, there are good reps and there are bad reps. The <u>best</u> reps will be your biggest ally. The poorly-trained, unprofessional rep will be your biggest frustration.

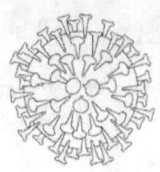

The Good Reps

Use your rep.

First of all, you might feel self-serving *using* somebody, but reps WANT to be used! A good rep is a resource; you can think of him/her as an extension of the product he/she sells. Their job is to get customers to understand the product – why it exists, what problem it solves, and how to correctly use it. A good product will be backed by science – reps will have all the scientific articles needed. Also, instructions-for-use, letters of interpretation and other documents can be sent by a rep, instead of having to frantically search for them on the internet and then wonder if what you found is even up-to-date. Often, they will be able to send them with the press of a few email buttons. A good rep is also connected and available during most working hours.

If you identify a need in your hospital – for example, let's say you want to implement a hand hygiene wipe for *patients* to use; a good rep can provide unbiased, evidence-based articles on his/her products so you don't have to spend hours doing literature reviews.

WIN-WIN Activities

There are certain ventures which can be done with your sales rep which I like to call WIN-WIN activities. These are value-added services that the rep will help with, which will benefit your institution as well as benefit the rep.

As an example, think of a rep who sells surgical site dressings. She has an initiative whereby she brings in a clinical specialist…usually a nurse who works for the surgical site dressing company. This specialist would meet with you and have you pull a list from your Electronic Health Record of all the patients that day who had surgical site dressings. You and the clinical specialist would then go around to each patient and collect data on the dressing integrity. Some questions you would want answered would be:

- Is the dressing clean, dry, intact?
- Is the dressing put on correctly?
- Is there tape, gauze, or other extra material?
- Is the dressing dated, initialed (according to your facility's policies)?

This data would then be compiled by the company's specialist. If you are working in a healthcare network and have several hospitals, this could be replicated at each location. The data could be provided as a simple Excel spreadsheet. This data would be a *snapshot of the gaps* in each unit of each hospital you visited. The "WIN-WIN" would be:

- Your facility wins because nurse leaders know what gaps to work on and look for to promote patient safety, quality improvement, and infection prevention compliance.
- The dressing company wins because they're ensured that their product is being used correctly and hopefully gaps are being fixed –

which would otherwise lead to infection and a possibility of blaming the infection on the product they sell.

A good sales rep can be used in other ways, too. Let's say a Joint Commission auditor comes to your facility. After complimenting your facility and saying what a good, clean place you have (as is often done on day one) they begin to visit areas (late in day one, into day two)…picking up items and asking questions that you have never thought about. Right around 9:30a.m. on day two, they visit your cardiac rehab area and find a disposable blood pressure cuff. A nurse is asked if this cuff is used once and thrown away, or if it's used on *more than one* patient. She responds with the truth – that it is used on multiple patients, cleaned between them, and discarded at the end of the day.

The Joint Commission auditor asks the nurse leader for two things:

1. Manufacturer's instructions-for-use (IFU) on the appropriate cleaning product for this blood pressure cuff – to verify that the disinfectant the nurse uses is compatible with the device.

2. Proof that the cuff is *rated to be used more than once,* or on more than one patient.

You have until noon to get this material to the auditor.

What's your next step? You could scour the internet for the information and you may find it – but the document you find may be outdated or for a different model of BP cuff. Also, many companies do not hire Infection Preventionists to write their IFUs, so the information on how to clean may not be practical. For example, it may say to clean the disposable cuff with a mild detergent and warm water.

Really?

So a better choice would be to send an email to your rep! Remember that right now you're reading the "Good Rep" section of this book. A good rep will be plugged in to his/her device and will either respond, or "c.c." someone else to respond. A good rep will also know the importance of being <u>timely</u> during a Joint Commission audit. The rep will have documents which tell all the minute, seemingly-trivial details such as how many times a disposable blood pressure cuff was "tested to" to determine its longevity. Also, he/she will be able to answer in a more practical way how to clean the cuff and whether your disinfectant is compatible with the cuff.

Remember that the rep wants to protect the relationship between your facility and his/her company. Providing documents such as these is one way the rep is prepared to continue this endeavor.

One psychological aspect you must possess when being audited is <u>power</u>, but it must be power under control. This method of leveraging others to get all of the items you need is a great way to invoke that power and be an effective leader. Often you will find that people are eager to help, especially if it is people with whom you have a business relationship. There is nothing unethical about leveraging these people to help you when you truly need something.

NOTE: Yes, you can use a disposable product more than once! The Resources section at the end of this book has a link to a great white-paper from Joint Commission International.)

.

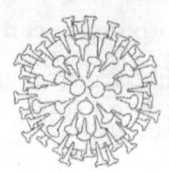

Bad reps

Those familiar with past books by this author know that there is a heavy emphasis on psychological principles and the human behavior aspect of Infection Prevention. The material in this book is no different. Understanding human behavior uncovers the "why"; it is especially handy as we begin to unravel the workings of sales reps. Ineffective reps may keep trying to sell the hospital a product that it doesn't want; some reps may have a poor product that lacks solid scientific basis, while other reps may struggle with boundaries and choose to not leave staff alone.

One tactic that is often used is the *"you'll be surprised!"* mentality. Here, the rep – instead of telling you about how the product can help you – resorts to telling you to do generic things that are so far off-base that you may not be ready for a rebuttal – for example, "go tell your I.T. department to pull numbers of patients who have phlebitis…you'll be surprised how many there are!". These little random details which aren't even in-line with how your facility operates are perfect for catching you off-guard as the rep tries to establish authority.

There is a psychological basis for this tactic. It is one of the <u>48 Laws of Power</u>, a book by Robert Greene. (It will be linked in the Resources section). This law says, "stir up the waters to catch fish". And in this sense, a person who may try unethical tactics to get people to buy new products is simply trying to confuse you. In the midst of this confusion, you begin to believe there is an HAI problem.

Though you may begin to see right through the intentions of this person (and you most-likely will after reading this book) it's important to leave emotion out of any communication that you might have with the rep – no matter how annoyed you may be. This person is still a *person*. Think of the person as having kids who call him/her "mommy" or "daddy". These reps are *people*. This rep may be early in his or her career and still learning to balance aggressiveness with stoicism. Also, reps sometimes move around; if you burn a bridge out of frustration with another person, and that person moves into a different company where they are now working with you, you will have an awkward situation.

So, in order to properly understand the inner workings of the mind of a sales rep, let's delve into the psychological aspects therein.

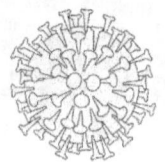

Sales Rep Psychology

In this chapter, we will discuss some tactics that good <u>and</u> bad reps will use. The tactics are used purposefully. It is important to learn about these so that you can expect and recognize when they're being used, and for what purpose.

Name Dropping:

As you're getting to know a sales rep, expect that they will mention people who are in power at your organization. They do their homework!! They may casually say, "yeah I have a meeting with (president of hospital)" or "I gave a presentation to (Vice President of Supply Chain/Contracts)". While these may be true, it is worth knowing that the art of remembering and regurgitating names is a technique that is used to accomplish the following:

1. **Name-dropping is supposed to make you feel more comfortable.** A sales person knows there's a chance that you don't have buying power in your organization, but you still may be able to help him/her get product pushed into the facility. If he/she can get you comfortable and become your "friend", then it's easier to talk to you about the new product that he or she is selling. It makes his/her job easier.

2. **Name-dropping is a way of establishing authority**. Similar to the point above, but a bit different; you'll notice that the rep never name-drops that he/she talked to the volunteer lady at the front desk or a random nurse on 2 East. Instead, the names mentioned are people who are easily-recognizable leaders. The rep is banking on you knowing the person whose name is being dropped, which will subconsciously get you to equate the rep's status with the leader's status.

YOUR BEST RESPONSE: There are a few things that you should do to correctly respond once you start hearing names of your organization's leaders come from a stranger's mouth…

a. Understand what's going on. Know that the rep is trying to get you to accept him/her. There's a *possibility* that the rep is trying to establish superiority over you if he/she mentions several names. But generally, and more-commonly, he/she is just trying to get you comfortable and out of the stranger-zone.

b. Ignore the names. Don't show any element of surprise in your facial gestures. Think of it like this: a rep had a meeting with a person who works at your work. The meeting may have gone well, but maybe it went poorly… or maybe neutral. Chances are, if it had gone well for the rep, you would know about it, as a new product would be coming in. (See Appendix A and Appendix B at the end of this book for guides on Product Review and Product Implementation). Even if you do want to get their product and do want the hospital to conduct business with him/her, the executives' names they mention are usually irrelevant. If you want to test what they're saying, you could always take down the name of the leader and say you'll check in with the leader to see what was covered in the meeting.

c. Beware of fishing! By this, I mean, sometimes an aggressive rep will want more names of people that he/she can call. If you mention additional people, you had better believe that rep will be remembering / writing down the names. And the next thing you know, he/she will be calling the names you mentioned and your name will be the one they drop!

How would you like for this stranger to call your vice president and say, "Hi there! I had a meeting with your Infection Preventionist (using your name) and he/she told me to call you to tell you about this new product which can clean better than your current one and blah blah blah"?

The Vice President will have <u>you</u> to thank for the rep's phone call. Don't respond with alternative names. You can be equally effective in your communication if you respond with job titles. Say things like, "you bring up some good points – I will talk to the surgical director about that."

Many years ago I was asked to be on a call with a rep with whom we had already determined we were not going to do business. I supposed that, for the purposes of being amiable, we weren't willing to just blow him off. So I was on the call and listening to his sales pitch, answering really generically whenever he'd ask questions. The rep had already dropped several names and their impressive job titles (which he got much of the nomenclature wrong). When I said I would talk with the director of the department, he literally said, "Oh yeah! I know them. What's his or her name again – isn't it "Tom?"". It wasn't anything close to, "Tom". Needless to say, I brushed right over that question!

3. The third reason a rep would use name-dropping is, ironically, so they may use your name in a legitimate way (contrast to the example earlier). Think of it this way: you are a subject-matter expert - an expert in your field of Infection Prevention. Your name carries weight in your organization. If you were a sales rep, wouldn't you like experts on whatever team you are creating? It was once said, by someone way smarter than me, that things are created twice: the first time it is created in the person's mind. Well, if a rep wants to create an actual team at your business for their product's implementation, the rep first creates it is in his/her mind. And now you are on the team. If conversations go well, he/she will use your name and will use the fact that you and the rep had a good conversation. Be prepared for your name to be dropped!

It is important to note that the above points are not necessarily bad things. If the product is truly a need of the hospital and most people want it, then the above points are important steps which need to happen in order for the product to become assimilated. The purpose for including these points isn't because you need to "watch out" for them. The above methods are tools. Tools used for implementation science. Tools used for sales. Tools used for change. When you are able to recognize them and know what they are and how each are used, you become more powerful, because now they cannot be used against you. "Knowledge is power"…isn't that what they say? And that is the point of this, and the other books; to give the Infection Preventionist the power to flourish in his or her career.

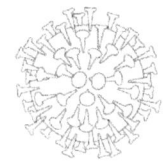

Contracts

Make friends with your contracts manager. This person can go by different job titles, but is a leader who deals with assigning contracts or accounts to vendors and is a person who leads supply chain. The point being that having a professional work-friend who can help you with product-related issues is an invaluable resource. As reps figure out your name, email, and phone, you will begin to have a steady stream of people calling you to tell you about the latest device that will revolutionize Infection Prevention in your hospital!

It is important to seek to understand how products are supposed to come in to your organization, with the intention that you will develop enough of a partnership to be comfortable telling the representative whether or not the hospital will entertain hearing more about their products. Perhaps, more appropriately, though, this could be done by the contracts manager. What would strengthen that process is if there was a good strategy in-place to get a new product into the facility. If each department or unit is able to order whatever they want and use it however they want, that is not a good, controlled use of money or product.

Think of the facility you're in as a huge wooden ship like the Titanic. Actually, the Titanic sunk…so think of your facility as though it is the Nina, Pinta, or Santa Maria. If each nursing unit or other 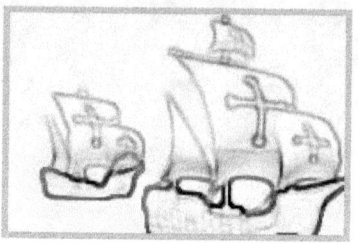 department can order whatever they want, whenever, from whomever, think of all those orders as holes being punched into the side of your ship. The ship could start to sink as costs are not in control, waste is not controlled, product confusion could be at an all-time high – and infections can result if products are being used improperly. Having a single "hole" that all products come in is much more controllable. This should be the Supply Chain department. They are the gatekeepers and will explain the process to the reps trying to get into the "ship".

Assuming your hospital is involved in the contractual purchasing of most products, the contracts manager can be your source to tell you if a product is on contract. Sometimes a product that comes to market is so different that there's nothing else like it. If it's something you want, then this is a good thing: you won't break any contractual obligation trying to get it in the doors. Other times, it is too similar to a product that's already on contract. In that case, it becomes much harder to get this new product. But that also means it can be easier to say, "no" to a rep – it would be breaking a preexisting agreement with another company and that can mean lots of money in penalties, etc..

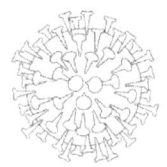

Processes v.s. Products

As the Infection Preventionist, the facility looks to YOU to be the subject-matter expert in all things "Infection Prevention". Yes it's everyone's job to follow IP procedures, but, going back to the last analogy, you are the one steering the ship for IP issues. Everyone else is on-board under your direction. A large part of your job as it relates to contracts is to be on the lookout for people who want to solve <u>process</u> problems with <u>products</u>.

Again – your job is to make sure people are not trying to use fancy new products to solve problems which are the result of poor processes. For example, if your facility wants to move from your Biopatch brand CHG sponge because you're having a higher incidence of CLABSI, but that sponge is often applied upside-down or placed on TOP of a dressing, and it's done by someone who has terrible aseptic technique, the problem isn't the Biopatch. Be certain that your back-to-basics are in-line before trying to get an expensive new product. This might mean meeting with leaders, auditing, implementing just culture/just-in-time coaching, developing tools, and/or using your educators to retrain clinicians. See the book "The Psychology of Infection Prevention" for more detailed information on how to go about finding gaps in practice, and what responses to expect when you go looking for them. (That book will be linked in a section at the end of this book).

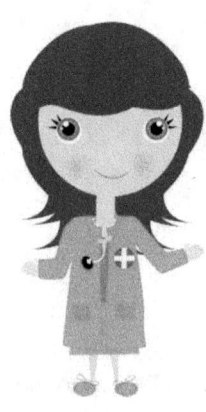

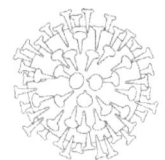

Trials

Ok, so imagine for a minute that there's a product that nurses want. You as an IP are in full-approval of this product being in-place and your Supply Chain manager wants this product because it'll save money. What is the next step? Well, it may need to be trialed. A trial is a period of time wherein a controlled group of people try the product and give quantitative and/or qualitative feedback.

In a healthcare setting it's recommended that trials last at least seven days so that opinions of weekday and weekend staff can be captured. These opinions are usually captured on a form called an "Evaluation Form". Names aren't important, usually, but items that are captured are generally the following: Job Title, Unit, quality of the item, ease of use, how it helps workflow, complaints, and if clinicians want this item for everyday use. There may be other questions you'd want to ask as well.

See the attachments section for a template that can be used (though you may have to copy/paste or re-create it).

Also, trials should not exist in a vacuum – that is, make sure different people are involved, or at least notified. Be specific as to what each person's job is, even if it's nothing. For leaders, it may be that they should expect a shipment of product on a certain day, and to put it in a certain place – or delegate someone to do that. For an executive, it could be a simple FYI memo stating that a product is being trialed (dates, unit, etc). Make sure you say, "no action is needed on your part" so they understand it's an FYI only. Create your group of people (email group or in-person). Consider involving:

Environmental Services leader

Nursing unit leader

Supply Chain leader

Nursing operations Director

Nursing executive (Vice President, Nursing or Chief Nursing Officer)

There may be others as you deem appropriate. Give clear instruction to everyone as far as when the trial will start, who will be receiving product, what they're supposed to do with the product, the reason for the trial, what evaluation forms to expect, where they send the forms, when the trial ends, and who to contact for questions. In the middle of the trial send a message asking how it's going. When it ends, send a third message stating so, and a reminder to send in evaluation forms. Once you tabulate everyone's responses, you will get a feel for how well the product has been received. This data should be communicated to the group. Then there should be a formal recommendation to the Supply Chain manager as to whether or not to get the product. Those are the basic steps for a trial.

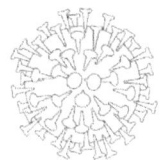

Guide: Re-using disposable products

Disposable products are meant to be thrown away.

It's that simple.

Or is it? A clinician may ask questions like:

- Does this mean it can be used only once?

- Can it be used multiple times on only one patient?

- What's the difference between "disposable", "single-use", and "single-patient"?

- Can it be used for one day and then disposed? What about one week?

None of the answers to these questions are obvious, but this guide will help.

1. First, determine what kind of "re-use" is being questioned. Look toward the Spaulding classification:

   a. Does the device touch only unbroken skin, such as a blood pressure cuff? (Non-critical).

   b. Does the device come into contact with mucous membranes? (Semi-critical).

   c. Does the device enter into sterile cavities such as blood vessels or organ spaces? (Critical).

This will determine the type of "re-use" that is being considered and the type of response needed to stay in compliance with patient safety regulations.

2. For items which are "Critical" or "Semi-Critical", a third-party company which is registered with the United States Food and Drug Administration (FDA) will need to take your used devices and completely reprocess and rebuild them. This is outside of the scope of this lesson, but just know that if any single-use critical or semi-critical devices are being re-used in your facility, that should raise a red flag in your mind.

3. For non-critical devices, like blood-pressure cuffs, there is a bit more flexibility for re-using the product a few times before its disposal.

Auditors will want to know:

- How many uses has the device been "tested to"? When the manufacturer is creating a disposable device, they will take an item or items out of a batch and use it over-and-over to determine how quickly it will wear out. If, for example, your device is tested to "at least 100 uses", you are able to say that this can be used 100 times or less before it is discarded. Most departments are not going to log how many times a disposable device is used, so, depending on patient load, they may re-use a device for a full day or week, and then dispose it. It's easier to prove to an auditor that they do not have 100 patients in a day or week, so they are in compliance.

How to get that information:

1. Ask your sales representative. Tell him/her that your facility is doing short-term re-use and need to know this information. It can be provided to you in the form of a letter from the company.

2. Go to the company's website. Sometimes there are downloadable resources such as "documents", "Instructions for use", or "Specifications" / "Spec sheets".

3. Calling the customer service number to the company can also work, as the associate may be able to email or fax the needed letter or document.

If you choose to re-use these non-critical products, be sure to have all documents accessible for audit-time. Also, any staff should be able to speak to the practice set forth in the clinic (such as the example of throwing the cuff away at the end of the day, or end of patient stay).

Auditors will also want to know:

- How are you cleaning the product? Sometimes the device's Instructions for Use (IFU) will be vague. Things that typically can be disinfected can have an IFU that says, "Use warm water and a mild detergent". If you are unable to find practical directions for disinfecting the product, ask the sales representative or the manufacturer. They may not tell you exactly what product to use, but they will at least tell you whether or not your hospital-approved disinfectant is suitable for use. Getting this in writing on their letterhead is a great step toward being able to re-use your disposable product.

*What about single-use drugs? Check out the book **DIP** in the Resource section.*

Resources

1. Check out the following link to read a great article on the re-use of single-use devices. It is a complex topic with lots of rules, but the Joint Commission International has done a great job of summarizing the rules and risks associated with this practice. https://www.jointcommissioninternational.org/assets/3/7/JCI_White_Paper_Reuse_of_Single_Use_Devices2.pdf

2. The Psychology of Infection Prevention. Here is a book on how changing mindset in your organization can help with lowering HAI. It's not as far-fetched as it may sound, and all ideas are backed by leaders in psychology. https://amzn.to/2O8GYrQ

3. Corrugated Care. When you're done getting the "Fancy New Products" unpacked, what are you going to do with all that cardboard? This book goes into detail on how to deal with cardboard in the hospital setting: https://amzn.to/355AFeW

4. 48 Laws of Power by Robert Greene: https://amzn.to/2MI4GsQ

5. DIP – Dental Infection Prevention. The Dental Professional's Guide to Infection Prevention Competency. https://amzn.to/2pZB7LF

These links go to products on Amazon, with whom the author affiliates. Amazon often pays a small stipend for sending business over, but it never costs the buyer any money. If you choose to look at these recommended materials, thank you.

IP Practice Questions - Test

1. Supply chain introduces a new product meant to be used for only a small portion of the hospital. However, no controls are in place for purchasing. This can lead to:
   a. Contracts
   b. Product creep
   c. Increase in HAI
   d. Lower costs

2. The Joint Commission just sent a team of auditors to your facility. They are asking detailed questions about a device that was implemented about a year ago. No one knows the exact answers but the auditors expect answers soon. Your best bet is:
   a. Guess
   b. Create a policy, procedure, or tip sheet and pretend you've always had this document
   c. Accept the finding and just try to do better at the next triennial visit
   d. Call the sales representative or company

3. Choose all that apply. Name dropping:
   a. Establishes authority
   b. Enhances familiarity
   c. Defines people on a new team
   d. Is used by good reps and not-so-good reps

4. In the past four months, *C. difficile* infection has increased significantly in your facility. You are not confident that the Environmental Services staff are competent enough to perform terminal cleans. Choose the worst three ideas:

    a. Pharmacy wants to add a few extra medications on the formulary to treat *C. difficile* differently

    b. Nursing wants to bring in a rep to talk about a better fecal collection device even though it isn't on contract

    c. Lack of training and competency verification should be escalated formally to the Vice President, Operations of the facility so change can be implemented ASAP.

    d. *C. difficile* should be treated empirically to lessen burden on the laboratory and so infections don't have to be reported to NHSN.

5. Why trial a product before bringing it into the facility?

    a. To make sure it's a good fit for the staff

    b. To collect qualitative and quantitative data

    c. To see if it will break a contract

    d. A & B

6. Reusing products that are supposed to be disposable is ok.

    a. It *can* be ok if you have documents showing how many times the product is tested to and know how to decontaminate & disinfect the product appropriately.

    b. Reprocessing and reusing disposable *critical* devices is a much bigger deal than with non-critical devices.

    c. Having information on-record from the manufacturer, and having your product representative on "speed-dial" will help you get through an audit more smoothly.

    d. All of the above.

7. It is best-practice to be "friends" with your supply manager because...

    a. He will be cleaning patient rooms.

    b. She will be unpacking all the cardboard, which is an infection risk.

    c. The manager will help you with standardizing products, which is good practice for saving your facility money and reducing product variability (which can prevent HAI).

    d. The product/supply manager often gets samples from vendors and can help you distribute them to clinicians.

8. Product trials should last at least five days so that weekday and weekend shifts can evaluate the product and give feedback

    a. True

    b. False

9. Products which are to be implemented to try to reduce HAI rates will probably need to be evaluated for months to get valuable statistical data

    a. True

    b. False

10. To be a high-achieving Infection Preventionist, you can't just rely on textbook knowledge – it's important to develop understanding of human behavior, psychology, and "soft skills' to deal with people and figure out their intentions.

    a. True

    b. False

Answers: 1c, 2d, 3abc&d, 4ab&d, 5d, 6d, 7c, 8b, 9a, 10a.

APPENDIX A: Product Review – Value Analysis

Objectives

1. Learn the fundamentals of Value Analysis

2. Understand the importance of an interdisciplinary team as it relates to Value Analysis

3. Through the use of this worksheet, develop and gain a framework for creating a Value Analysis plan.

The first thing an organization must do to avoid variability and confusion is to standardize the process of bringing in new products for trial or permanent implementation.

If products are not reviewed by a group of people before being offered for use in the healthcare setting, there will be cost issues, legal issues, patient safety and satisfaction issues, and effects on staff and healthcare workers.

Risk Analysis

Standardization

List the product and its purpose and cost:

List products within the organization that this will currently replace:

List out any Patient Safety Impacts:

Staff/Healthcare Worker Impacts:

Infection Prevention & Control Impacts:

Patient Satisfaction Impacts:

Staff Satisfaction Impacts:

Cost Impacts:

Are these outcomes measureable – to see if it's making a difference?

  If YES, they should be measured:

- The person responsible for measuring baseline and end-outcomes is:_____

- The date range for measurement is:_____ through _____.

- How will it be measured?

- Where will this data be presented? (Committees, meetings councils, etc)

- How will this data be presented? (Graphs, slideshow, presentation, etc)

The ability to obtain certain products is sometimes influenced by how well the product is doing in the market. Because of this, there should be plans in place for certain circumstances. It is important to make sure the following are in place:

Procedure for:

- Product recall – Why was the recall done? If for a patient/life safety issue, is there a procedure for removing this item and prohibiting staff from ordering it? How will its absence affect patient care? How fast can alternative product come in?

- Emergent use – This can stem from the above question – if it is a matter of patient safety or a patient's life, can a product be rushed through the process faster than the ordinary process? What counts as emergent use?

- Product discontinuation- What happens when the product is no longer available? Will another be substituted? Will there be a gap in availability?

ALGORITHM:

Healthcare Worker (HCW) REQUEST – fills out "Product Request Form". The HCW signing this form becomes the champion/owner of the request and will lead, delegate, and be responsible for any product trial. This person will pull in education.

The person requesting the product should fill this out – he or she is the champion.

PRODUCT REQUEST FORM

Requestor Name & Contact Info:

Delegate Name & Contact Info (if applicable):

- Trial Request
- Full Product-Implementation Request
- Emergent Use Request

Product Manufacturer, Name, and Description:

Projected Rate of Usage:_____

Reason for Request (Include Science-Based Articles here)

Sales   Representative   Name,   Contact   Information   and
Company:_____ _____

Circle All That Apply:

This Product Is:

FDA approved

Latex-free

Consumable/Disposable

Capital equipment

Needing installation

Involving:

    o Clinical engineering

    o Facilities management

    o Infection Prevention/Control

    o Employee Health

    o Others?

Requestor Signature:_____

Date Submitted:_____

Contract Type:

Contract #_____

CONTRACT MGR. REVIEW:

❏ Accepted

❏Rejected

Reason Rejected: _____

Requestor notified by: _____

❑   Forwarded   to   committee   for   review   on   (date)

_____

COMMITTEE ACTION:

❑ Approved by (TBD) Committee and/or Contract Manager on (date)

_____

❑ Reason for Rejection:

_____

Signature:_____

Date:_____

The Product Request Form goes to the contract manager who will either approve or deny.

If the contract manager does not approve of this product, a decision will need to be made for your organization whether or not any type of appeal process can be done to have someone take a second look.

If approved – Contract Manager sends to applicable departments (which are identified on the Product Request form)

A group of people from the organization will need to come together to make decisions about what products to trial, which ones to bring into the organization permanently, and which to deny. This multidisciplinary group should represent all aspects of the organization, as each has a different, but equally-important reasoning for having interest in product acquisition. Below is a list of representation which would typically be on this type of committee.

At this point, some decisions should be made regarding the committee, including:

o How often does the committee meet?

o When are vendors brought in or included?

o How involved should vendors be?

The Product Request From then goes to the New Product / Value Analysis Committee.

New Product / Value Analysis Committee: Infection Prevention/Control, Employee Health, Environmental Health and Safety, Facilities, Clinical Engineering, Nurse Leadership, Contract Manager, Product Champion, VP Supply Chain/Contracts, Education, Finance, Custodial Services

The Committee will either deny, or approve. If approve – it can be either a Product Rollout or a Trial.

• If Trial:

o Fill out "New Trial Worksheet" form (see Appendix A)

o Vendors are expected to provide products at no cost for 30 to 60 days.

o For trials longer than 30 – 60 days – pricing and ordering expectations should be determined beforehand.

o Need process written for having departments ordering products after 30-60 days.

• If Product Rollout:

o Fill out "New Product Implementation" form (See Appendix B)

o Define exactly what has to happen to get a new product an order number.

▪ Who is involved?

▪ What information needs to be provided from whom and to whom to get the order number and to get products on each shelf in each unit.

o How long do products have to be ordered v.s. when can they be automatically stocked? Often times, supply chain departments like to have usage data for a few months before they automatically begin stocking products.

This ends the process of Product Review and Value Analysis. From here, product is brought to the organization's facility / facilities and staff is educated on it according to the organization's education procedure. Sales representatives often are on-site providing this education as well.

APPENDIX B – New Product-Trial Worksheet

Product:

Hospital(s) or Other Clinical Location:

Champion(s) at Each Location:

Contact Information for Champions:

Length of Trial:

Date Range:

Product Request Form Completed?   yes   no

Quantity of Product Needed

Product Sales Representative:

Contact Information for Product Sales Rep:

STATUS:
Date

APPENDIX C: New Product Implementation Form

Product:

Hospital(s)

Champion(s) at Each Location:

Contact Information for Champions:

Product Request Form Completed?   yes   no

Quantity of Product Needed

Product Sales Representative:

Contact Information for Product Sales Rep:

Organization Education Representative:

Education Contact Information:

STATUS:

Date   Notes

You could put a picture of the product or logo at the top, here.

APPENDIX D: Evaluation Form

Trial: Blah Blah Product – **Date Range:**_____

Hospital/Unit:

Job Title/Credentials (Circle One): RN   MD Other:_____

	Strongly Disagree	Disagree	Neutral	Agree	Strongly Agree
Was this product easy to use / convenient?	O	O	O	O	O
Was the product good quality?	O	O	O	O	O
Did the product help workflow?	O	O	O	O	O
Other items you want to capture could be entered here	O	O	O	O	O
I support the use of this item as an every-day product for our unit or hospital.	O	O	O	O	O

Comments:

www.ingramcontent.com/pod-product-compliance
Lightning Source LLC
Chambersburg PA
CBHW070842220526
45466CB00002B/854

* 9 7 8 1 6 9 9 9 9 4 2 2 2 2 *